#2 IN THE SERIES OF BOOKS YOU'LL ACTUALLY READ

Health +
Healing
& Essential Oils

ANDREW EDWIN JENKINS

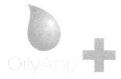

OilyApp +

A BOOK YOU'LL ACTUALLY READ ABOUT THE "OILS OF ANCIENT SCRPITURE""

Health + Healing & Essential Oils: A Book You'll Actually Read About the "Oils of Ancient Scripture." Copyright 2019, Andrew Edwin Jenkins

ISBN number = 9781793007360

Adapted from *Supernatural Healing, Super Practical Health, Oils of the Bible, and You!* Copyright 2018, Overflow, LLC. And, adapted from *The Field Guide to Healing-* Copyright 2016, Overflow, LLC. All right reserved. No part of this book may be reproduced in any form or by any means without permission in writing by the publisher. ISBN 13: 978-1985144262, ISBN 10: 1985144263

Connect online!

Podcast-
OilyApp.com

Social-
www.Facebook.com/OilyApp
www.Facebook.com/OilyApp
www.Instagram.com/OilyApp

YouTube-
www.YouTube.com/Overflow

Website-
OilyApp.com
Jenkins.tv

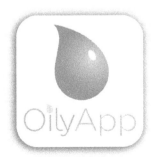

Contents

AN OVERVIEW OF WHERE WE'RE HEADED!

Introduction	5
1. Designed for Health	9
2. Health & Healing	15
3. Anointing	31
4. The Oils of the Ancient Scripture	57
*Next Steps	71
*OilyApp+	75

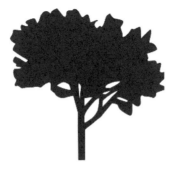

Introduction

ABOUT THIS BOOK + ABOUT THIS SERIES

We created OilyApp (go to OilyApp.com to learn more) with the goal of educating you about Young Living's vast array of incredible products. The app is uniquely the only third party app that's an approved partner of. Young Living Essential Oils, passing a strict compliance review each time we update.

OilyApp works well with Young Living's stated mission of taking oils into every home in the world. Once the oils get there, people need to know… *how do we use them?!*

Whereas shipping a desk reference to everyone is cumbersome and difficult (besides, who wants to always lug it around!?), most people have a smart phone. And, books can't do stock notifications, manage your personal inventory, or update anytime a new product is released.

An app is the perfect solution.

Furthermore, the app was created by actual members (Ernie Yarbrough, one of the founders, and his wife are Royal Crown Diamonds). In other words, it was built in the field for use in the field.

The next thing

After a few years of providing users with OilyApp, it became apparent that another addition was needed for product users and business builders who wanted to go to the "next level." Enter OilyApp+, a web-based experience designed to provide users with more relevant information- things like scripts they could use to learn and/or educate their teams, graphics that were relevant and educational, and access to Diamond+ leaders.

We created OilyApp+ in less than two weeks from its conception.

From the beginning, we knew we wanted the OA+ to include video courses and online scripts- tools you could use to review and then teach your "people" what you were learning.

After a few weeks, the thought hit us: *What if we made the scripts into small books, too- small pocket-sized books people could easily review and use to study, to lead others, and even to teach classes?*

Hence the title you have in your hand.

The script and the videos where we teach the material are available in OA+ (access it all at OilyApp.com).

About this book —->>> Health + Healing + Oils

That leads us to the subject of this book.

INTRODUCTION

In this book (and the videos) we talk about miracles and prayer and natural health- all in the same sitting. Some people think that to choose one is to negate the other- or vice versa. We've learned each of these things work together.

You'll find this book to be super-informative, as well as ultra-practical. And, we pull stories straight out of the Bible and show you the oils they used- and why…

We'll also show you things like...

- The guy most likely to talk about the power of the Holy Spirit (Luke) was also a doctor. And, the guy who healed a ton of people (Paul), also taught people how to be well…

- When Jesus sent the disciples out, He didn't just empower them to perform miracles, He also showed them to teach people how to be + live well.

And, we'll discuss rarely-talked about topics like anointing, laying on of hands, and other things we often overlook.

Want to know more?

Flip the page. Join us on the journey!

Defining the terms

Throughout this class, for simplicity sake...

- *Healing* refers to something God does, something supernatural

- *Health* refers to something we do, to choices we make

We'll see that both of these actually work together.

1. Designed for Health

YOU WERE CREATED TO LIVE WELL + BE WELL

"...ON EITHER SIDE OF THE RIVER WAS THE TREE OF LIFE, BEARING TWELVE KINDS OF FRUIT, YIELDING ITS FRUIT EVERY MONTH; AND THE LEAVES OF THE TREE WERE FOR THE HEALING OF THE NATIONS" (REVELATION 22:2 NIV).

1. When we see healing manifest on earth, we're actually seeing Heaven coming down, breaking into the world in which we live.

- Jesus told the disciples to tell people the Kingdom of God had come near when they healed them (Matthew 10:7, Luke 10:9).

- He Himself said that when He drove out demons, **it was a sign that the Kingdom was present** (Matthew 12:28, Luke 11:20).

2. The prophet Ezekiel & the apostle John learned something interesting when they saw the Tree of Life in Heaven.

- "On each side of the river stood the tree of life... **And the leaves of the tree are for the healing of the nations"** (Revelation 22:2 NIV).[1]

- "Fruit trees of all kinds will grow on both banks of the river. Their leaves will not wither, nor will their fruit fail. Every month they will bear fruit, because the water from the sanctuary flows to them. **Their fruit will serve for food and their leaves for healing"** (Ezekiel 47:12 NIV).

- Whereas most people think about the tree of life- and its presence in Heaven- in *symbolic* terms, simply *spiritualizing* it, we need to remember that **the first time we see the tree in Genesis it is an actual tree in the physical world.** Adam and Eve could have eaten its fruit. They could have climbed this tree or sat in its shade. It wasn't symbolic; it was *real.*

---

[1] The word for "healing" here is *therapeuo.* We'll learn more about the word later. For now, think about this: *Why is there healing in Heaven?*

3. Healing & wholeness were present in the beginning, before sin. Health & wellness were not results of the chaos created by the fall. Healing & wholeness already existed.

- **A moment ago I suggested healing shows us the presence of the future.** That is, we see healing in the book of Revelation.

- **Healing also shows us the reality of our past.**

4. In Eden, God gave every plant for food- and more!

- Genesis 1:29-30 reads, "Then God said, 'I give you every seed-bearing plant on the face of the whole earth and every tree that has fruit with seed in it. **They will be yours for food.** And to all the beasts of the earth and all the birds in the sky and all the creatures that move along the ground—everything that has the breath of life in it—I give every green plant for food.' And it was so" (NIV).

- **The Hebrew word used here, which we translate as "food," is** *oklah.*[2]

  - *Oklah* includes the things you eat, but it is more. *Oklah* includes medicines. Notice, these were here in the beginning.

---

2 The Old Testament was originally penned in Hebrew.

- We see the same word used in Ezekiel 47:12 (see the previous page). The word *oklah*, in both instances, would include herbs, teas, and other plant-based products.

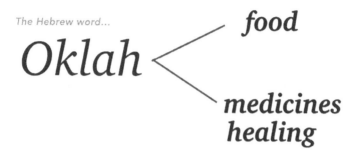

The Hebrew word...

Oklah < *food* / *medicines healing*

- **"...the plant kingdom offers countless varieties of medicines created by God-sufficient to address every ailment known to humankind.** Instead of spending billions on secular profit-motivated research to create new synthetic drugs, antibiotics, vaccines, and surgical procedures, our research should be towards discovering, studying, and applying the vast array of medicines that God has already perfected in forms already available to us."[3]

- **"Let your food be your medicine and your medicine be your food"** (Hippocrates).

---

[3] David Stewart, *Healing Oils of the Bible*, p165.

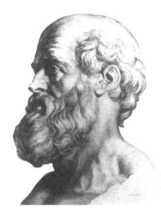

"

LET YOUR FOOD BE
YOUR MEDICINE AND
YOUR MEDICINE BE
YOUR FOOD...

— Hippocrates

"

5. Why was healing & wholeness available in the Garden before sin (especially if sickness is a result of the Fall)? And why is it present in Heaven?

- **We were created to *choose* wellness, just like we were created to *choose* intimacy.** In fact, I believe we will want to choose wellness when we walk fully in who we were designed by God to be.

- **"God's perfect will is not to heal you; His perfect will is that you don't get sick."**[4]

- **There are different kinds of healing, as we will see.** We often look *only* at "instant" healing as a valid form of the kingdom's in-breaking. But, we'll see that *choosing* to

---

[4] Dr. Henry Wright, *A More Excellent Way*, p12.

1. DESIGNED FOR HEALTH

walk a pattern of health and wholeness is a valid form of healing as well- and was used by the Apostle Paul and even Jesus. In fact, Jesus commissioned His disciples to take this form of healing to others.

- In other words, **we were created to walk in healing, to experience health, and to enjoy the physical world around us**.

- **Our health should incorporate each part of our person: body, soul, and spirit.** We're created for *total* wellness. So, we shouldn't just limit health to our physical bodies, as we often do. Or, on the other extreme, limit health to our spirit.

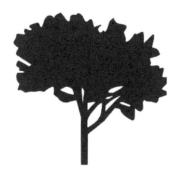

2. Health & Healing

BOTH DEMONSTRATE GOD'S DESIGN FOR US

"BELOVED, I PRAY THAT YOU MAY PROSPER IN ALL THINGS AND BE IN HEALTH, JUST AS YOUR SOUL PROSPERS" (3 JOHN 2).

"WHO FORGIVES ALL YOUR INIQUITIES, WHO HEALS ALL YOUR DISEASES" (PSALM 103:3).

1. There are foundational concepts we should believe about healing.

- In this chapter we will see that **healing is broader than we often think.**

- **Healing can happen instantly- or "over time."** It can happen as what we might refer to as a *miracle*, or as a series of healthy choices and habits we choose to embrace.

- **Healing involves the total person- not just the physical body.** And, in fact, most healing will happens from the "inside out," as the spirit (the part of us that is one with God) and the soul (our mind, emotions, etc.) are addressed. When this happens, many times the physical symptoms simply disappear.[5]

2. Three different words refer to "healing" in the New Testament. Let's introduce two of them here.

- **Understanding why different are words used is important as we begin a healing ministry- or even as we seek healing.**

- **Here are two of the Greek words (the New Testament was**

> UNDERSTANDING WHY THERE ARE DIFFERENT WORDS USED IS IMPORTANT AS WE SEEK HEALTH & HEALING.

---

[5] I've seen dozens of people healed simply by forgiving someone. In addition, I've seen many people healed when they receive a revelation of their identity as a beloved child of a loving Heavenly Father.

originally written in Greek and Aramaic) for *healing*.[6]

- *Iaomai*- means "miraculous" and "instantaneous" healing. This is how we most often envision Jesus healing, though this word only appears 30 times in the New Testament. (See examples in Matthew 8:13, Mark 5:29, Luke 8:47, John 12:40.)

- *Therapeuo*- means "to serve, to attend to, or to wait upon menially" and "to heal gradually over time with care." This word appears 40 times in the Bible- a bit more than the instant cures we usually associate with miracles. (Matthew 4:23-24, Mark 1:34, Mark 6:13, Luke 5:15, Acts 5:16, Acts 8:7, Revelation 22:2.)

3. I believe in- and have seen- "iaomai" (healing)- firsthand.

- My brother gouged an eye when he was younger. He was never supposed to be able to see. Today, **his eye is completely whole and has been for over 35 years. He's in his 40s and still doesn't even need glasses. That's *iaomai*.**

- My sister had a severe heart murmur when she was a small child. My parent's took her to a specialist in Houston who charted the arrhythmia. My Dad prayed and then took her back a few weeks later. The physician asked if

---

6 The discussion on the two Greek words comes from David Stewart's *Healing Oils of the Bible*. See p91.

they could use the new chart side-by-side in his classes with the old chart- one to show what a sick heart looked like on paper and the other to show what a perfect heart looked like. **They still use that chart 30-plus years later. Again, that's *iaomai*.**

- My uncle died twice at UAB. He came back. Twice. They didn't pump, aggressively resuscitate, or shock him. **The doctor walked to the waiting room both times and said, "Another miracle." That was over 15 years ago. Another *iaomai*.**

4. I also believe Jesus uses "therapeuo," that is, "natural means of health" over time.

- Yes, I believe Jesus heals people in the moment. I also believe He can do things in other ways, too. Specifically, **I believe He can use natural means over time in the same way that He also uses medical professionals and miracles. It's *all* His healing, anyway.**

- **Now, we would say that *all* of Jesus' healings in the Bible were miracles.** None of us would make a list and say this one doesn't count, that one was normal, that one was something else… This wouldn't be up for debate!

- **Yet, one of the words for "healing" that is used in the Gospels clearly shows us that Jesus didn't *always* heal immediately.** Sometimes, He administered a series of instantaneous healings and other times He likely "taught people to be well."

- The word *therapeuo*, another word translated in English as "healing," appears significantly *more* times than *iaomai*, showing us there might actually be a slight emphasis here.

Two Words for Healing

	APPEARS	MEANING	HAPPENS
IAOMAI	30 times	Instantaneous healing	Spontaneously, in the moment
THERAPEUO	40 times	To serve, to attend to, or to wait upon menially- teaching them to be well	Intentionally, over time

5. Both types of healing happen in harmony with one another throughout Jesus' ministry.

- **Matthew 8 illustrates this healing spectrum.** Specifically, the stories in this chapter tell us "how" Jesus heals people. We will look at each of these instances and make a few more observations about healing in general. We will see both types of healing.

2. HEALTH & HEALING

- **First, we see that Jesus absolutely heals instantly**. In one of His first miracles, Jesus goes to Peter's house.

  - There, we see Peter's mother-in-law is ill with a fever. Remarkably, Jesus touches her hand, the fever leaves her, and she serves them dinner (8:15). He heals her in a moment.[7]

  - This is an example of *iaomai*- just like my brother, my sister, and my uncle.

- **Second, we see that Jesus often teaches people to be well.** Word travels quickly about Peter's mother-in-law, and the townspeople began flocking to the house. Here's how it reads: "When evening came, many who were demon-possessed were brought to him, and He drove out the spirits with a word and healed all the sick" (Matthew 8:16, NIV).

  - Matthew 8:16 tells us that everyone in the town who is demon-possessed and sick is brought to Jesus. **He heals *all* of them**, according to the Bible (8:16).[8]

  - The phrase "with a word... healed all who were sick..." literally means, according to most Bible

---

[7] She was probably deathly ill- this wasn't just a case of "higher-than-normal temperature." She was on her deathbed, I believe.

[8] Here's the tension today: Why aren't *all* people healed now? Clearly some are not healed. And, Psalm 103:3 tells us that our Father heals all of our diseases and forgives all of our sins. Both. To the same degree. Completely. Since our reality doesn't match what we see in the Bible, we've shifted to "disease management" rather than trying to understand why "all" aren't healed of "all" things. We're no longer looking for a cure- and prevention. This is odd because we don't question whether or not He forgives all sin!

commentators that I've checked, *"He taught them to be well"* (8:16).

- Want to guess what Greek word is used there in the New Testament? That's right, *therapeuo*, the second word for healing.

iaomai **"**

15 HE TOUCHED HER HAND AND THE FEVER LEFT HER, AND SHE GOT UP AND BEGAN TO WAIT ON HIM.

therapeuo

16 WHEN EVENING CAME, MANY WHO WERE DEMON-POSSESSED WERE BROUGHT TO HIM, AND HE DROVE OUT THE SPIRITS WITH A WORD AND HEALED ALL THE SICK. **"He taught them to be well"**

"

6. We see both types of healing in the Apostle Paul's ministry, too.

- Acts 28:7-9 tell us that he healed Chief Publius, who was on his death bed, sick with dysentery. **The Bible details that Paul *iaomai* him.** He instantly made him well.

- The remainder of the islanders gather to the hut, much in the same way that the crowds flocked to Jesus after He healed Peter's mother-in-law. Luke, a physician who is traveling with Paul, explains that **Paul then *therapeuo* the entire island.** That is, he taught them how to live well.

"

PAUL WENT IN TO SEE HIM AND, AFTER PRAYER,
PLACED HIS HANDS ON HIM AND HEALED HIM.
iaomai
9 WHEN THIS HAD HAPPENED, THE REST OF THE
SICK ON THE ISLAND CAME AND WERE CURED.
therapeuo

— Acts 28:8-9 NIV

"

7. Here's what it means that Jesus heals in two kinds of ways…

- Sometimes, Jesus heals instantly. Other times, He teaches people how to be well.

What it means…

IAOMAI	THERAPEUO
HEAL LUNG CANCER	Teach ills of smoking
CURE DIABETES	Show how to eat better
HEAL STDs	Display beauty of true intimacy
HEAL PHYSICAL NUISANCES	Give directions on being alive!

2. HEALTH & HEALING

- Make note, **sometimes Jesus touches us and we are** *dramatically* **changed in that moment. Other times, He imparts His wisdom to us so that we** *can* **be changed.**[9]

- **Think about what this really means:**

  - Jesus can heal lung cancer- but *He can also teach us about the ills of smoking.*

  - He can cure diabetes- *He also shows us how to eat better.*

  - He can heal us of sexually transmitted diseases. Also, *He provides us with directions on how to live whole and healthy lives, as well as experience the joy of true intimacy.*

---

[9] In John 5, we read the story of Jesus healing the man who sat paralyzed by the Pool of Bethesda. You probably know the story fairly well. He has been sick for 38 years. As such, he has gathered in a place where many sick people gather. They all believed that whoever jumped into the pool first, when the waters stirred, would be healed. He had likely seen people healed because he explained to Jesus that he had no one to push him in when the waters stir.

"Someone always jumps in ahead of me," he said, excusing his condition.

Jesus asked if he actually wanted to be well. The man offered excuses as to why he could not be. In spite of the man's reservations, Jesus healed the man. Notice that He didn't lay hands on the man; He simply commanded him to gather his things and walk! That is clearly *iaomai*.

Here's an oddity: **we later read that the man didn't even know it was Jesus that healed him,** because he's not certain who Jesus even is! The man begins walking and is instantly bombarded by the religious leaders. They chide him for carrying his mat on the Sabbath. A bit later, Jesus runs into the man (who, again, doesn't even know who Jesus is), telling him "go and sin no more, lest something worse happen to you" (worse than a 38-year illness!).

Here's where I think the concept of *therapeuo* comes into play here: The man received an instant healing, an *iaomai*. Now, though, he must walk in health and wholeness or he can become sick again. In other words, *therapeuo* and *iaomai* are not opposed to each other- they always complement and enhance.

- *He* can heal us of the dozens of physical nuisances that we've grown to tolerate. *Or, we can take His directions and experience what it really means to be alive!*

Sometimes, Healing Comes as You Walk it Out

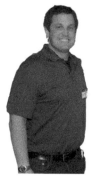

Unwellness- Many of the issues I faced were a direct result of the lifestyle I was living.

DOWN 50 POUNDS!

Wellness- I experienced two kinds of healing as I began living intentionally.

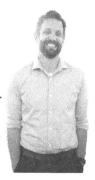

- **In the same way that I've seen *iaomai*, I've also experienced *therapeuo*.**

  - A few years ago, I was 50 pounds overweight.

  - Some of the symptoms I had included:

    - Low energy levels

    - I couldn't sleep well at night (Oddly enough, I could crash on the couch in the middle of the afternoon fine, however)

2. HEALTH & HEALING

- Digestive issues (blood in my stool, regularly; daily bouts with diarrhea)

- Shortness of breath- even though I was exercising regularly

- Creaking bones- and hardly able to walk- if I woke up in the middle of the night or when I woke up first thing in the morning

- Constant need to urinate during the night (led to sleepless nights)

- Inability to lose weight- regardless of my activity level

- I made the decision to walk in wellness (*therapeuo*).

- Some breakthroughs happened instantly.

  - I slept through the night immediately- and the snoring was gone.

  - My digestion issues all improved instantly- I believe it was an example of *iaomai*.

- Other victories came as I continued walking in wellness, "walking out" my healing.

  - Energy levels increased- and continued increasing

  - I became stronger and stronger physically

- My thinking became much sharper
- Muscle and joint pain quickly diminished

- **You might be "healed as you go," too- just like I was *and* like the ten lepers were who encountered Jesus** (see Luke 17:12-19).[10] Or like Naaman the leper in the Old Testament, who was healed instantly (2 Kings 5).[11] What's the difference? It's all His healing, anyway! To experience *therapeuo* there is almost always an associated action!

8. We were designed to choose life, to live well.

- It's interesting that the leaves which bring healing are seen in the Garden *before* sin entered the equation (Genesis 1:29) as well as *after* the effects of sin are resolved (see Revelation 22:2).

  - *Why were there leaves for healing in the Garden of Eden, before sin entered the equation?*

---

[10] It has been my experience that people are often healed "gradually," as they walk in obedience. *They reap more of the Kingdom harvest as they sow more into the principles of the Kingdom.* For instance, think about the ten lepers that were healed as they obeyed Jesus, walking to show themselves to the priests (and presumably to offer the required Levitical sacrifices) (Luke 17:14). In some instances, we see both of these methods of healing working together: the power for the healing is given immediately, but people must appropriate it by walking in the healing.

[11] Yes, on outward change could have happened instantly. God had the power to do this. But, I believe God was more interested in using this situation to deal with Naaman's pride. Now, this doesn't mean that God caused the leprosy to happen. However, Naaman was a better man afterwards because he was physically well and he had dealt with the heart issue of pride. In the same way, I'm better and more disciplined, having walked through the healing process rather than just having an instantaneous health change.

- *Why do we see leaves "for healing" in Heaven, where there's no more death & dying or sin?*[12] My thought: total health is our destiny. So, health now shows us a snapshot- even if a dim one- of our future.

- **It seems that walking in health and wholeness is a choice- in the same way that walking in intimacy is a choice.**

  - Adam & Eve chose to walk in relationship with their Heavenly Father. They were not "robots" without a free will.

  - Might they also have chosen to walk in health and wellness? And aren't those choices- intimacy with our Father and walking in wellness- that we must make even now?

Remember our definitions...

Healing **refers to something God does, something supernatural.**

Health **refers to something we do, to choices we make.**

---

12 Genesis 1:29: ""I give you every seed-bearing plant on the face of the whole earth and every tree that has fruit with seed in it. They will be yours for [*oklah*]." Remember, *oklah* is food and medicines. These existed in the beginning before sin. I initially thought God was already making provision for sin. However, Revelation 22:2 shows us that the tree of life has an interesting function: "...On each side of the river stood the tree of life, bearing twelve crops of fruit, yielding its fruit every month. And the leaves of the tree are for *the healing of the nations*" (emphasis added). Notice, healing properties exist in Heaven- even though there is no sin there. The word used in Revelation 22:2 is *therapeuo*, by the way.

9. The Church is called to preach the Gospel of the Kingdom, which we now see is broader than the forgiveness of sins.

- **Jesus commanded His disciples- *and empowered them*- to preach the Gospel of the Kingdom when He sent them out. And, He told them to heal as they did** (Luke 9:2, for example).[13]

- **Notice the "kind" of healing He sends them to demonstrate and teach:**

  - When Jesus sends out the 70, He says: "Heal the sick there, and say to them, 'The Kingdom of God has come near...'" (Luke 10:9). The word He uses is *therapeuo*. They weren't just to instantly heal people (which we know they did from other places throughout the New Testament). They were told to teach a Kingdom way of life.

  - Notably, this is the same way He sent the 12 in Luke 9:1-2. He "gave them power and authority over all demons, and to cure diseases." These two actions- *physical healing and spiritual deliverance*- were part of the complete salvation / *sozo* we just saw. Notably, "He sent them to preach the Kingdom... and to *therapeuo* the sick" at the same time" (NKJV). Instant healing and "healing over time" aren't at odds.

---

[13] They had to receive the healing, first- and then take it to others.

2. HEALTH & HEALING

- We see this same dynamic happening in other
  Gospels. Matthew writes that Jesus told them,
  "Heal the sick, cleanse the lepers, raise the
  dead, cast out demons..." (Matthew 10:8 NKJV).
  Matthew says that Jesus said to *therapeuo* the
  sick... even while raising the dead and spiritually
  freeing the oppressed. Instant healing (*iaomai*)
  and healing over time (*therapeuo*) are present.

2. HEALTH & HEALING

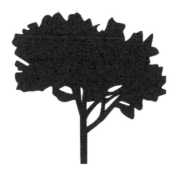

3. Anointing

LAYING ON OF HANDS WAS SIGNIFICANT IN BIBLICAL TIMES

"AND THESE SIGNS WILL FOLLOW THOSE WHO BELIEVE: IN MY NAME THEY WILL CAST OUT DEMONS; THEY WILL SPEAK WITH NEW TONGUES; THEY WILL TAKE UP SERPENTS; AND IF THEY DRINK ANYTHING DEADLY, IT WILL BY NO MEANS HURT THEM; THEY WILL LAY HANDS ON THE SICK, AND THEY WILL RECOVER" (MARK 16:17-18 NKJV).

"IS ANYONE AMONG YOU SICK? LET HIM CALL FOR THE ELDERS OF THE CHURCH, AND LET THEM PRAY OVER HIM, ANOINTING HIM WITH OIL IN THE NAME OF THE LORD. AND THE PRAYER OF FAITH WILL SAVE THE SICK,

AND THE LORD WILL RAISE HIM UP" (JAMES 5:14-15 NKJV).

"SO THEY WENT OUT AND PREACHED THAT PEOPLE SHOULD REPENT. AND THEY CAST OUT MANY DEMONS, AND ANOINTED WITH OIL MANY WHO WERE SICK, AND HEALED THEM" (MARK 6:12-13 NKJV).

1. We see essential oils throughout the Scripture.

- **Essential oils are an integral part of the healing ministry in the Scriptures.** We have as much detail about the oils as we do about baptism, the Lord's Supper, and some other fundamental practices in our faith.

- Yet, in our Western culture of allopathic care, we often miss this one![14]

2. The tree of life and the trees in the Garden of Eden were full of the power to nurture health.

- See the Intro, the explanation of *oklah* as "foods and medicines." **The first time God gave plants to man, He was giving food *and healing.***

---

[14] Allopathic care = western medicine. It consists primarily of disease treatment rather than prevention. It leans heavily on medicines, pharmaceuticals, interventions, etc., as opposed to lifestyle changes and natural approaches.

- The "law of first mention" is a Bible study principle that means that anytime we see something in Scripture, we should **look to the first time it appears to see how we should interpret it.** This, should effect how we view the world around us.

> ESSENTIAL OILS ARE AN INTEGRAL PART OF THE HEALING MINISTRY IN THE SCRIPTURES.

- **Plants aren't just food; they are healing.**

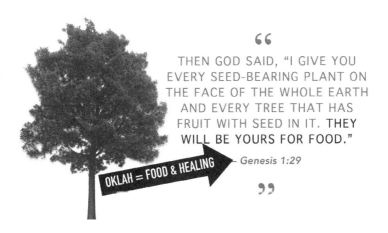

66

THEN GOD SAID, "I GIVE YOU EVERY SEED-BEARING PLANT ON THE FACE OF THE WHOLE EARTH AND EVERY TREE THAT HAS FRUIT WITH SEED IN IT. **THEY WILL BE YOURS FOR FOOD."**

– Genesis 1:29

99

OKLAH = FOOD & HEALING

3. The healing properties of plants have been used throughout history. Many cultures have been using them since Creation.

> **"**
> ANCIENT TEXTS AND HISTORICAL AND
> ARCHAEOLOGICAL EVIDENCE- INCLUDING
> EGYPTIAN HIEROGLYPHICS, CHINESE
> MANUSCRIPTS, GREEK PHYSICIANS' RECORDS,
> AND BIBLICAL REFERENCES- SUGGEST THAT
> ESSENTIAL OILS HAVE BEEN AN INTEGRAL PART
> OF HEALTH AND WELLNESS FOR CENTURIES.
>
> — *Scott Johnson*
> *Surviving When Modern Medicine Fails*
> **"**

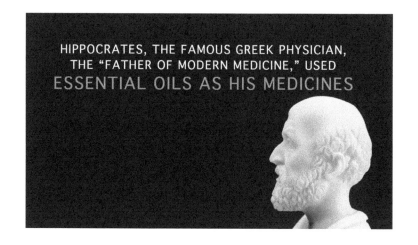

HIPPOCRATES, THE FAMOUS GREEK PHYSICIAN,
THE "FATHER OF MODERN MEDICINE," USED
ESSENTIAL OILS AS HIS MEDICINES

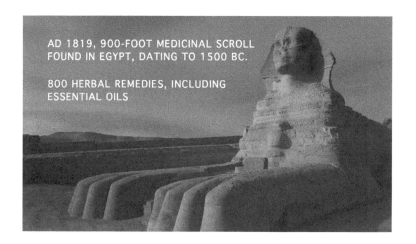

AD 1819, 900-FOOT MEDICINAL SCROLL FOUND IN EGYPT, DATING TO 1500 BC.

800 HERBAL REMEDIES, INCLUDING ESSENTIAL OILS

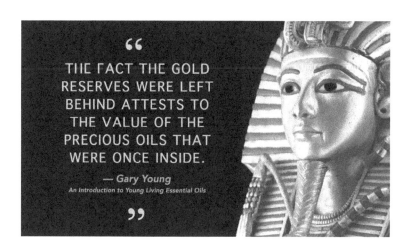

"

THE FACT THE GOLD RESERVES WERE LEFT BEHIND ATTESTS TO THE VALUE OF THE PRECIOUS OILS THAT WERE ONCE INSIDE.

— *Gary Young*
An Introduction to Young Living Essential Oils

"

3. ANOINTING

- "Ancient texts and historical and archaeological evidence-including Egyptian hieroglyphics, Chinese manuscripts, Greek physicians' records, and Biblical references-suggest that **essential oils have been an integral part of health and wellness for centuries.**"[15]

- **Hippocrates, a famous Greek physician, used essential oils as his medicines.**

- 1819, **a 900-foot long papyrus was found in Egypt, dating to 1500 BC. It is believed to be a "medicinal scroll,"** and contains over 800 herbal prescriptions and remedies as well as references to essential oils.[16]

- 1922, King Tut's tomb was discovered. The crew which explored the tomb found 50 alabaster jars (which would have held 7 liters of oil each, for a total of 350 liters total). Raiders had taken the oil but left the gold behind. **"The fact the gold reserves were left behind attests to the value of the precious oils that were once inside."**[17]

- **"Kings would barter and buy land, gold, and slaves with their crudely extracted oils, because they were more valuable than gold."**[18]

---

[15] Scott Johnson, *Surviving When Modern Medicine Fails*, p8.

[16] Gary Young, *An Introduction to Young Living Essential Oils*, p3.

[17] Gary Young, *An Introduction to Young Living Essential Oils*, p3.

[18] Gary Young, *An Introduction to Young Living Essential Oils*, p3.

The OLD TESTAMENT

Essential oils appear 200x

Central to the Tabernacle

Priests anointed with a specific blend

4. From Egypt to the Tabernacle and through the Old Testament, essential oils prove central to what God was doing.

- **There are 200 references to essential oils in the Old Testament alone.**[19]

- One of the big focal points of the Old Testament is the Tabernacle.[20] **God gave specific instructions about the Tabernacle and even the oils used in it.** The Lord gave very specific instructions, also, about the building of the Tabernacle, the furniture and relics that were to be placed inside, and the adornment of the priests who would administer specific sacrifices.

---

[19] Review Dr. Stewart's book *Healing Oils of the Bible* for a detailed overview.

[20] Particularly in the time of Moses, we see the prominence of essential oils. There are well over 200 references. The Egyptian connection makes sense when you remember that Moses was steeped in Egyptian tradition. He was a true "prince of Egypt" and raised as such, until he fled for his life after killing a fellow Egyptian in the fields.

- He was clear, too, that **those priests were to be anointed with a** *specific* **blend of essential oils which He relayed to Moses:**

    - "Take the finest spices: of liquid myrrh 500 shekels, and of sweet-smelling cinnamon half as much, that is, 250, and 250 of aromatic cane, and 500 of cassia, according to the shekel of the sanctuary, and a hin of olive oil. And you shall make of these a sacred anointing oil blended as by the perfumer; it shall be a holy anointing oil" (Exodus 30:23-25, ESV).

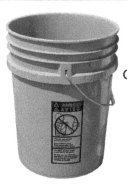

The Anointing Oil

MYRRH   1 gallon (500 shekels)

CINNAMON   1/2 gallon (250 shekels)

CALAMUS   1/2 gallon (250 shekels)

CASSIA   1 gallon (500 shekels)

OLIVE OIL   1 & 1/3 gallons (a hin)

- 500 shekels is about one gallon.[21] In effect, Moses was blending the following:

    - Myrrh- 1 gallon (500 shekels)

    - Cinnamon- 1/2 gallon (250 shekels)

---

[21] See *Essential Oils Pocket Reference*, pp6-7.

3. ANOINTING

- Calamus- 1/2 gallon (250 shekels)

- Cassia- 1 gallon (500 shekels)

- Olive oil- about 1 & 1/3 gallons ("a hin" is slightly larger)

- When complete, he had the equivalent of a *five gallon bucket* of anointing oil. If they didn't ration it when applying the anointing oil, it would *drench* the man being anointed.

> **"**
>
> BEHOLD, HOW GOOD AND PLEASANT IT WHEN BROTHERS DWELL IN UNITY!
>
> IT IS LIKE THE PRECIOUS OIL ON THE HEAD, RUNNING DOWN ON THE BEARD, ON THE BEARD OF AARON, RUNNING DOWN ON THE COLLAR OF HIS ROBES!
>
> IT IS LIKE THE DEW OF HERMON, WHICH FALLS ON THE MOUNTAINS OF ZION! FOR THERE THE LORD HAS COMMANDED THE BLESSING,
>
> LIFE FOREVERMORE.
>
> — *Psalm 133:1-3 (ESV)*
>
> **"**

- Consider the passage above Psalm 133:1-3 (ESV).

- Notice that the oil flows down the robes as it falls off the priest's head, fills his beard, and hits the collar. **That's a *lot* of oil!**

- **Some people in the Tabernacle had the specific job of maintaining the oil.** They were known as "perfumers" (see 1 Chronicles 9:30, Nehemiah 3:8).

> **ESSENTIAL OILS ARE AN INTEGRAL PART OF THE HEALING MINISTRY IN THE SCRIPTURES.**

- We read that the incense of the Temple was of a sweet smell (see Exodus 30:25f.). Notably, it was common in those days for public areas to have essential oils diffusing throughout the building. The Romans cleansed public buildings with them (we will see that oils can purify things as well as people). In other words, **essential oils were in common use culturally.**[22]

"FRANKINCENSE IS GOOD FOR EVERYTHING FROM HEAD TO TOE."

— Ancient Egyptian Proverb

5. We even see essential oils in Jesus' life and ministry.

---

[22] *Essential Oils Pocket Reference*, p5.

3. ANOINTING

- Jesus' additional name, Christ- or *Christos*- means "anointed one."[23] When priests and kings were set into office, they were anointed with essential oils.[24] And, they were put in place for a specific purpose. Of course, Jesus came to *save*, which we discussed earlier.[25]

- At His birth, **the magi brought Gold, Frankincense, and Myrrh. Notably, two of the three items are essential oils.** The ancients believed Frankincense had great healing properties- it was common for doctor and healers to carry both Frankincense and Myrrh with them.[26]

> CHRIST- OR CHRISTOS- MEANS "ANOINTED ONE." WHEN PRIESTS AND KINGS WERE SET INTO OFFICE, THEY WERE ANOINTED WITH ESSENTIAL OILS.

  - "Myrrh is still recognized for its ability to help with infections of the skin and throat and to rejuvenate tissue. Because of its effectiveness in preventing

---

23 In Acts 10:38 we read: "...how God anointed Jesus of Nazareth with the Holy Spirit and with power, who went about doing good and healing all who were oppressed by the devil, for God was with Him" (NKJV).

24 When was Jesus anointed? We read that He was anointed by a woman of the street multiple times- including at the beginning of His ministry and at the end, preparing Him for the Cross (see Luke 7:36f and Mark 14:3f.). These instances are at the homes of two different men, and they happen at two different times. Since these are from two of the "synoptic Gospels" we can presume they are following a similar timeline of Jesus' life. The two writers simply record two different events.

25 See the discussion on the word *sozo* (chapter 2- Habit 1: Think, B., 9.).

26 Consider what you would bring to a king if you could bring anything of great value?

bacteria growth, myrrh was also used for embalming."[27]

- Did Jesus use Myrrh with the lepers? Given the fact that many traveling healers in the day would have had both Frankincense and Myrrh with them at all times, it seems plausible to think so.

- Does this make the Bible stories less dramatic, less supernatural? *Not at all.* If anything, it makes the experience of these truths more accessible. Face it, sometimes *iaomai* seems out of reach; *therapeuo* is always at hand, however.[28]

- **When Jesus sent His disciples out, He sent them to heal-** *while laying their hands on people with oils.*

  - Mark 6:7-13 records perhaps the first instance of this: "And He called the twelve to Himself, and began to send them out two by two, and gave them power over unclean spirits… And they cast out many demons, *and anointed with oil* many who were sick, and healed them" (NKJV emphasis added).

  - Jesus' younger brother, James, gives the same instructions to early church leaders: "Is anyone among you sick? Let him call for the elders of the church, and let them pray over him, *anointing*

---

[27] *Essential Oils Pocket Reference*, p5.

[28] And, as we discussed earlier, even when a miracle comes, you maintain the healing by walking in *therapeuo*.

him with oil in the name of the Lord" (James 5:14 emphasis mine).

- **It seems that the oils were legitimate, full strength oils- not symbolic oils.**

  > FACE IT, SOMETIMES IAOMAI SEEMS OUT OF REACH; THERAPEUO IS ALWAYS AT HAND, HOWEVER.

  Remember, when Jesus was anointed with Spikenard, the argument was related to the cost (see Mark 14:1-9, Matthew 26:1-13). The oil used to anoint Him was worth a year's wages of a common laborer. We will discuss the importance of the quality of the oils used in a moment.

- **We known Jesus' body would have, historically speaking, been prepared for burial with oils, too.** Joseph of Arimathea and Nicodemus prepared Jesus' body for burial (John 19:39).[29] They needed a large quantity of essential oils do to this (about 100 liters- or 75-100 pounds). This would be worth about $150,000-$200,000 in today's retail environment, showing 1) their great wealth as well as 2) their great reverence for Jesus.

6. What's being assumed by the Gospel writers? A lot about several important subjects.

---

[29] You may remember that Jacob was buried in Genesis 50:26. According to the embalming customs of the Egyptians who buried him, his body would have been treated with such oils also. See *Healing Oils of the Bible*, p140.

3. ANOINTING

- **The authors of the Bible simply assume we know some the basics of essential oils.** There are hundreds of references throughout the Bible meaning the authors must have assumed we would know what was being referenced. The truth is that their *immediate* audience did know!

- **This is simply how they wrote- there are *many* predominant ideas that the authors of the Bible never explain, simply assuming we'll know what they're talking about.** For instance:

  - *Crucifixion*, the centerpiece of the New Testament- and the very act that most of the Old Testament points to- is never

> THERE ARE MANY PREDOMINANT IDEAS THAT THE AUTHORS OF THE BIBLE NEVER EXPLAIN, SIMPLY ASSUMING WE'LL KNOW WHAT THEY'RE TALKING ABOUT.

    explained. Yet, it remains the focal point of the Bible and, really, human history.

  - *Baptism* is never explained- hence, much of the disagreement throughout Church history as to the proper way to baptize someone.

  - *Communion*- or the "Lord's Supper"- isn't really explained in any detail, either. In fact, the way they practice communion in the Bible seems radically different than how we do it. They seem to celebrate with an entire meal (see 1 Corinthians 11).

3. ANOINTING

- *Anointing* appears throughout the Bible. Strangely, we don't see many details on this, either. (Incidentally, the act *never* seems symbolic in Scripture; it appears that something actually happens in the moment of the anointing, as well.)[30]

- Finally, **essential oils** appear in the Scripture hundreds of times.[31] Though someone living in Jesus' day would know what the authors meant when they referred to oils (or any of the other important concepts listed above- *crucifixion, baptism, communion, anointing*), we typically don't.

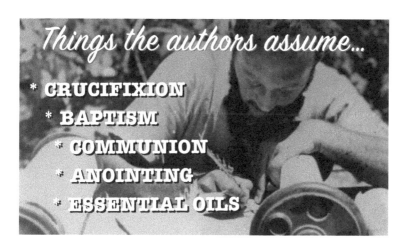

Things the authors assume...

* **CRUCIFIXION**
* **BAPTISM**
* **COMMUNION**
* **ANOINTING**
* **ESSENTIAL OILS**

---

[30] We've gotten so confused about this one that we've even changed the name to *ordination* in some church circles to just "start over" with a new concept.

[31] "The Bible contains 33 species and more than 500 references to essential oils and the aromatic plants from which they came" (Stewart, *Healing Oils of the Bible*, p7).

- **Some people may make the case that they didn't have doctors, then, so they relied more on natural means.**

  - It may be true that, partly. I think we actually rush to medical professionals today because of their easy access. If they weren't so accessible, we might take more responsibility for some of our health choices.

  - Oddly enough, "doctors" appears in the Bible *three* times (see Luke 2:46, Luke 5:17, and Acts 5:34).[32] In each instance, written by Luke (a physician, who would know what a *doctor* is), the reference is to "doctors of the law"- meaning *rabbis* or *teachers* as opposed to practitioners of healing.

  - Physicians were ordered to prepare Jacob's body for burial (Genesis 50:2). From this story, we learn that they were practitioners of essential oils. And, we see Luke repeatedly referring to the concept of *therapeuo*.[33] Perhaps there is a strong link here.

7. The healing power of touch... is both ancient and new.

_____

[32] *Healing Oils of the Bible*, p49.

[33] Remember, Luke (a doctor) is actually the most prolific author in the New Testament.

- Remember, Jesus touched the leper- even though He is able to (and does, throughout the New Testament) heal with just a word. **To a person who has experienced isolation, human touch is powerful.**

TOUCH
=ONE OF THE MOST POWERFUL HUMAN FORCES

- In fact, **modern science suggests human touch is one of the most powerful forces.**

    - "We come equipped with an ability to send and receive emotional signals solely [by touch]. In one experiment participants communicated eight distinct emotions- anger, fear, disgust, love, gratitude, sympathy, happiness, and sadness- with accuracy as high as 78 percent."[34]

    - "I have witnessed the power of healthy touch to heal, deliver, redeem, and restore people in mind, body, and spirit. Loving touch has the power to draw out the introverted autistic child, make an outcast teenager feel loved and accepted, or communicate safety to a battered

---

[34] "The Power of Touch,," by Rick Chillot, *Psychology Today*, published March 11, 2015.

woman. Healthy, loving touch reminds us of our God-given worth and identity."[35]

- "According to neuroscientists, our brains are programmed for touch."[36] The study cited in this article actually shows that "touchier teams" (i.e, basketball, football) performed better than less touchier teams. Apparently, something is communicated in the high-fives, the shoulder taps, and the fist bumps that is actually quantifiable.

- **Perhaps it makes more sense, now, that laying on of hands is almost always mentioned with healing** (this happens in other instances, too, when something powerful is happening, such as the declaration of a new identity or destiny). In fact, the laying on of hands- *touch*- is mentioned in several powerful ways throughout Scripture. Touch is so important that it's not just limited to healing.

- **Notice the times we see touch- i.e., "laying on of hands"- in the Bible.**

    1. *Healing-*

        - Mark 6:5 (Hands were laid on people- and they were healed.)

---

[35] "Have We Forgotten The Power of Touch?" by Nicole Watt, in *Christianity Today*, June 6, 2014.

[36] "Power of Touch a Transformative, Healing Force." See CBN News, CBN.com, September 8, 2014.

3. ANOINTING

- Mark 7:32 (People beg Jesus to lay hands on a man who is deaf and mute.)

- Mark 16:17-18 (Jesus says His followers will lay hands on the sick.)

- Luke 4:40 (Jesus laid hands on people who were brought to Him from throughout the village, even into the evening.)

2. *Imparting spiritual gifts / supernatural power to do something-*

- 1 Timothy 5:22 (Paul cautions Timothy not to lay hands on new leaders too soon; he actually imparts some power to them when he does.)

- 1 Timothy 4:14 (Gifts are imparted by the elders to others stepping into ministry roles- would this be like an anointing? Did it involve oils?)

- Deuteronomy 34:9 (Moses gives Joshua wisdom.)

3. *Blessing people-* Mark 10:16 (Jesus laid His hands on the children and blessed them.)

4. *Imparting the Holy Spirit-* Acts 8:17 (Peter and John laid hands on the Samaritans and the Holy Spirit was imparted to them.)

- **Question: Were these instances of "laying on of hands" simply instances when people were touched by** another? Or did they operate like times of an anointing (which we will discuss in a moment), instances where *more* than a simple touch occurred? Is James giving us details about laying on of hands (he includes oils) that would have been commonly practiced?

> DID THEY OPERATE LIKE TIMES OF AN ANOINTING... INSTANCES WHERE MORE THAN A SIMPLE TOUCH OCCURRED?

We know that when kings and priests were anointed, oils were used. We also know that when Jesus sent the disciples to lay hands on the sick, He instructed them to use oils. Was this the common practice for each of the verses above? Is this what we would expect to see if we were present in those instances? For the answer, let's take a deeper look at essential oils and how they are used.

LAYING ON OF HANDS

* **HEALING**

* **GIFTS / POWER**

* **BLESSING**

* **HOLY SPIRIT**

8. Oil quality matters, particularly when we understand what a Biblical anointing actually is.

- **Consider the touching and the oils involved in a Biblical anointing.**

  - The touch was more than a simple, light touch.

    - To *anoint* means "to rub" or "to smear."[37]

    - "... the Biblical references in Mark and James where healing take place with prayer, laying on of hands, and anointment with oils... the Biblical meaning of the word 'anoint' means 'to massage or rub with oil.'"[38]

    - In other words, the touch wasn't a simple touch any more than baptism means to "flick a little bit of water on someone" (*baptizo* means "to submerge").

    - This is an intimate sort of touching- thoroughly appropriate but *connecting*.

---

[37] *Healing Oils of the Bible*, p6.

[38] *Healing Oils of the Bible*, p xxiii.

ANOINT

"TO RUB" *-OR-* "TO SMEAR"

- An anointing of any type most often included a large amount of oil.

    - Remember the "excessive" amount of oil that flowed down the beard of the priests, per Psalm 133:2?

    - Remember the amount of oil used on Jesus, when the woman anointed Him (see Matthew 26:7, Mark 14:3)?

    - Remember that Jesus actually rubbed mud over a blind man's eyes when anointing him and laying hands on him (John 9:6)? It was enough dirt and substance to actually make mud...

- An anointing might happen on the head, on the shoulders, on the hands, or even the feet (as in the

> AN ANOINTING OF ANY TYPE MOST OFTEN INCLUDED A LARGE AMOUNT OF OIL.

instance of Jesus).[39]

- The touch, and the oil, would be noticeable to any bystanders.[40]

- **The smell would be predominant... so consider the role the limbic system plays in the process here.**

  - When you breathe, oil molecules move to the back passages of your nose, to the amygdala- the central headquarters of the limbic system. "The limbic system manages your storage for all of your emotional experiences."[41] This is why you can smell something- Fall leaves, apple pie, etc.- and a memory instantly arises in your soul. And, it's why hearing a certain song will instantly transport you back to a different time and place...

  - Notably, the limbic system responds to words, smells, sound... all sensory input- yet, it doesn't

---

[39] For those familiar with the technique, the "raindrop" could actually be called an anointing if married to Scripture and/or prayer.

[40] Various verses throughout the Bible show that the Holy Spirit covers people when He anoints them. In some way, the oil would be similar. See Psalm 2:2, Lamentations 4:20, Ezekiel 28:14, Habakkuk 3:13, Zechariah 4:14, Luke 4:18, Acts 4:27, Acts 10:38, 2 Corinthians 1:21, 1 John 2:27.

[41] *Healing Oils of the Bible*, p24.

have the capacity to communicate with
language.[42]

- In other words, **when anointing someone with oil, we
are doing far more than just "touching" them
physically.** We are:

  - *Expressing to them that they are important and
    loved- through touch.* And, now we understand
    that far more is communicated through touch
    than we might have imagined possible.[43]

  - *We are offering them something helpful for the
    body.*

  - And, this is before we have even prayed! *In the
    next step we will invite God's supernatural power
    to do it's work!*

  - In other words, this isn't a symbolic- any more
    than baptism, communion, and laying on of
    hands is symbolic. There is more happening than
    we see- and we expect physical results to
    manifest!

---

[42] A few more points about the limbic system: Dreams originate in the limbic system.
Spiritual understanding occurs in the limbic system- not the assessment of facts and
information, but revelation and intimacy. This is why it's difficult to sometimes communicate
an encounter you've had with the Lord- and why it "falls flat" when you try to explain it to
others. Words can't do it justice, because the limbic brain has such a greater capacity than
words (re: revelation), while simultaneously having no capacity for written or spoken
language.

[43] Review "the healing power of touch" earlier in the book.

NOT
SYMBOLIC
ACTUAL

* BAPTISM

* COMMUNION

* LAYING ON HANDS

* ANOINT TO HEAL

- Now, at this point, you might wonder: *Why not just pray?*

  - Prayer and oils- and other forms of *therapeuo-* actually work together and enhance each other. "Each

  > PRAYER AND OILS- AND OTHER FORMS OF THERAPEUO- ACTUALLY WORK TOGETHER AND ENHANCE EACH OTHER.

  increases the power of the other such that their combined ability to heal is greater than the sum of the two… When we pray over the oils, their frequencies increase."[44]

---

[44] *Healing Oils of the Bible*, p93.

ANOINTING INVOLVES < the power of touch

+

something useful for the body

4. The Oils of the Ancient Scripture

WHAT THEY DO + WHAT YOU NEED = DIRECTION TO GO

"...HE BEGAN TO SEND THEM OUT TWO BY TWO, AND GAVE THEM POWER... SO THEY WENT AND PREACHED... AND THEY CAST OUT MANY DEMONS, AND ANOINTED WITH OIL MANY WHO WERE SICK, AND HEALED THEM" (MARK 6:7,12,13 NKJV).

"YOU ANOINT MY HEAD WITH OIL" (PSALM 23:5 NIV).

4. THE OILS OF THE ANCIENT SCRIPTURE

1. Think about your body and what you need.

- Before we move through the oils, I want to do a quick exercise. **Take a moment and think about your body and your health and make a list of the areas where you would like to see greater wellness and support.**

- *Do you want to experience:*

    - *Improved digestion?*

    - *Immune system function?*

    - *Brain health?*

    - *Better sleep?*

    - *Improved mood?*

- Make a list of your top 3 priorities and keep it in mind while we are discussing the oils.

    - _____

    - _____

    - _____

2. Now, review the oils of ancient Scripture, making note of how any of these may support needs you- or someone you know- has. We'll walk through these in alphabetical order, for ease.

> ## *Covering 12 of 10 oils*
>
> Note: we'll cover Galbanum & Spikenard, which are featured throughout the Bible but are not in Young Living's Oils of Ancient Scripture kit. They may be purchased separately.

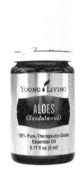

Aloes / Sandalwood is an oil of love.
Nicodemus took Sandalwood to prepare Jesus's body for burial, along with Myrrh (John 19:39). David writes of garments being scented with Sandalwood, making one glad (Psalm 45:8).

Some people suggest Sandalwood supports the immune system and the lymphatic system (the lymphatic system is the circulatory system, which is vital to the immune system).

Others suggest Sandalwood serves as an natural aphrodisiac- that it works as a great cologne for men or a natural support for the female reproductive system.

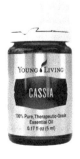

Cassia supports the immune system. Moses included this as an ingredient in the anointing oil for the priests (Exodus 30:22f.). This makes sense when we remember the priests would have handled animal sacrifice daily- and, hence, would have been exposed to their blood any uncleanness or disease they carried.

Also believed to be an anti-fungal, Cassia exudes uplifting feelings. In other words, it's believed that you emotionally feel the effects of the immune support.

We see this cleansing oil mentioned over 50 times throughout the Bible.

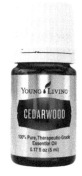

Cedarwood oil addresses the needs of the mind. The wooden beams in the temple were of this tree (1 Kings 4:33, Psalm 104:16). Mentioned 25-plus times throughout the Bible, Cedarwood supports clear thinking.

People have used Cedarwood to address symptoms of ADHD & ADD, as well as hair loss and sleep deprivation.

This oil stimulates the mind in a positive way, and is believed to also facilitate emotional cleansing and release.

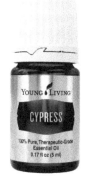

Cypress, in Greek, means "live forever." We learn from the Old Testament that the Temple featured Cypress in addition to Cedarwood (1 Kings 9:11).

The wood is strong and durable- the doors of St. Peter's Cathedral are constructed of Cypress and have been standing unblemished, with no signs of aging, for 1200 years. Perhaps this is why God instructed Noah to build the Ark from Cypress. Tradition says the Cross was Cypress, too, creating eternal salvation in the same way Noah's Ark facilitated temporal salvation.

Cypress may improve circulation, strengthen blood capillaries, and energize white blood cells.

Cypress may be diffused to ease feelings of loss, as well as bring a sense of accompanying emotional ease. In the Temple, Cedarwood assisted the head, while Cypress supported the heart!

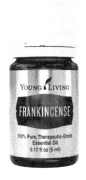

Perhaps the greatest use of Frankincense is spiritual alertness! Extracted from the Boswellia tree, the Biblical word "incense" is translated as *Frankincense*. So, many times when we read *incense* the author is likely referring to this oil.

Frankincense was used to anoint newborn sons of kings throughout the ancient world. The Egyptians believed it was good for "everything from gout to a broken head" (literally, "everything from head to toe"). This explains why many healers in Jesus' day would carry Frankincense with them.

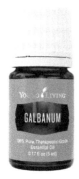

Galbanum exudes grace. In the same way that Jesus declared "I did not come to call the righteous, but sinners…" (Mark 2:17), Galbanum is an oil noted for its ability to address things that are broken or out of balance and bring restoration…

Galbanum has been known to address cramps, abscesses, indigestion, aches & pains, scars, and wrinkles. Galbanum also elevates the mood and helps a person feel whole and alive.

Perhaps this is why Galbum, as part of the Oil of Incense, was diffused in the Temple during the time of sacrifice. People would see- and sense- grace in action.

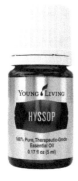

Hyssop means "Holy herb" in Hebrew. Holy means, "set aside for God's use."

Hyssop was believed to erase feelings of guilt and anxiety and bring about a feeling of one-ness with God. This is why David prayed to be cleansed with Hyssop after committing adultery and murder (Psalm 51:7).

Ancients also believed Hyssop could ward off evil spirits, horrible thoughts, and sinful feelings. Remember, the blood of the Passover lamb was smeared with Hyssop on the doorposts (Exodus

12:22), and Jesus was offered a drink while on the Cross with a Hyssop branch (John 19:29).

Hyssop was used to purify temples in the ancient world. This is amazing, considering the Scripture says you are now God's temple (1 Corinthians 6:19).

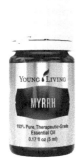

Myrrh was prized for its ability to support healthy skin. Ancients believed Myrrh helped the skin elude infections, that it helped reverse stretch marks after birth, and that it was emotionally uplifting at the same time. If Mary applied Myrrh to her skin, it would have soothed and calmed baby Jesus even while supporting her body.

Esther treated her body with Myrrh for 6 months in preparation for her night with the king (Esther 2:12). Including her story, we see Myrrh over 150 times in the Bible.

We see Myrrh in the Holy Incense (see Exodus 30:23,34). As "fixative" Myrrh helps other oils maintain their effects longer and stronger- which would help since the incense burned 24 hours a day.

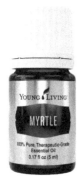

Myrtle is known for supporting the respiratory system- the throat, the lungs, the nose...

Singers in Solomon's temple are believed to have anointed their throats with Myrtle. Physicians now believe this would clear their vocal chords of mucus and allow for better air flow.

Incidentally, Esther's name is Myrtle (*Hadassah*), as her name was changed in the harem.

Isaiah 55:13 tells us that instead of thorns, Myrtle will grow. Instead of being choked out, God's people will be able to spiritually- and physically- breathe!

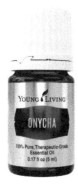

Onycha is a healing oil. Part of the anointing oil referenced in Exodus 30:34, Onycha was used to address open wounds, it was rubbed on the stomach to ease pains, and it was used to stimulate the senses.

This is a thicker oil that almost feels like a gel.

Rose of Sharon (Cistus) denotes peace, rest, and refuge. This oil comes from a large white flower found in the fertile plains between Jaffa and Mount Carmel in Israel (sometimes referred

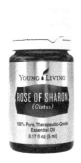

to as the Rose of Sharon). In other words, amidst the backdrop of a desert, it is an oasis.

Rose of Sharon may promote emotional health and bring a sense of emotional stability. As well, it may also promote physical stability throughout the body; people have been known to use Cistus to ease tremors and / or arthritis pains.

Solomon's wife proclaimed that she was his Rose of Sharon (Song of Solomon 2:1). She was his refuge, his oasis.

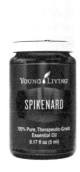

Spikenard reduces nervous tension and soothes. This is the oil used to anoint Jesus- at the beginning of His ministry and just before He faced the Cross (see John 12:3f. and Matthew 26:7f.). The oil reduces anxiety, eases feelings of nausea, and dissolves nervous tension.

Song of Solomon speaks of the table at his home smelling like Spikenard (1:12). Indeed, this oil was prized in the ancient world- remember the objection Judas had to the anointing was that the cost of the oil amounted to a year's wages!

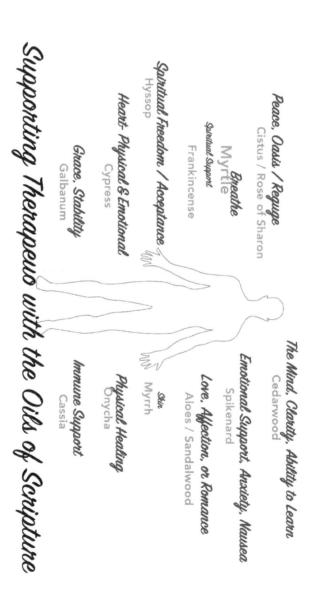

Supporting Therapeus with the Oils of Scripture

Peace, Oasis / Refuge
Cistus / Rose of Sharon

Breathe
Myrtle
Spiritual Support
Frankincense

Spiritual Freedom / Acceptance
Hyssop

Heart, Physical & Emotional
Cypress

Grace, Stability
Galbanum

The Mind, Clarity, Ability to Learn
Cedarwood

Emotional Support, Anxiety, Nausea
Spikenard

Love, Affection, or Romance
Aloes / Sandalwood

Skin
Myrrh

Physical Healing
Onycha

Immune Support
Cassia

3. Notice how the entire person is supported.

- Oils address the physical, emotional, and spiritual needs of the total person.

- God is concerned, then, with the entire person- *body, soul, and spirit.*

4. Pause and make notes of what you may need.

- _____

- _____

- _____

- _____

5. Once you understand the purposes of the oils, you'll probably begin recognizing them throughout the Bible.

- There are a few places we see the Oils of the Scripture *together*. Let's look at a few of those examples. You may study others on your own.

- For our purposes in this workbook we'll look at the Holy Incense (Exodus 30:34-36), the protocol for cleaning the lepers (Leviticus 14), and Jesus' birth.

HOLY INCENSE

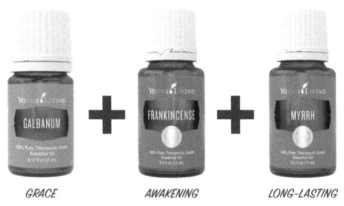

GRACE   AWAKENING   LONG-LASTING

OilyApp.com- for iOS + Android. Download for graphics + videos + a pocket reference on your phone. Young Living approved. 100% compliant, 200% awesome.

Notice how each of these oils "fit" together to make a perfect blend for the Temple. First, we see grace in action (Galbanum). And, we see the presence of healing (Onycha), along with spiritual awakening (Frankincense). This sounds a lot like sozo, the third word for healing we learned earlier. As well, Myrrh elevates and magnifies the qualities of all other oils, and is noted for its ability to bring peace and calm- to the body, soul, and spirit.

Remember, today, you are the temple (1 Corinthians 6:19). This is the same power-combo that resides in you- Grace, Healing, Spiritual Awakening, and Long-lasting Peace.

CLEANSING LEPERS

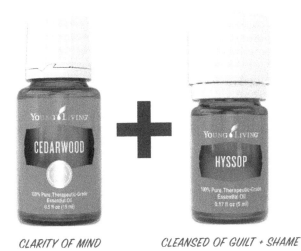

CLARITY OF MIND   *CLEANSED OF GUILT + SHAME*

OilyApp.com· for iOS + Android. Download for graphics + videos + a pocket reference on your phone. Young Living approved. 100% compliant, 200% awesome.

Notice two of the oils used to anoint lepers. We see they were given a renewed mind (Cedarwood), which would see reality differently. And, they were cleansed of the old guilt and shame associated with their disease (Hyssop). Many New Testament scholars believe leprosy is a "type" (read: foreshadowing) of sin- as sin separates us from others, it brings its unique stigma and condemnation, and it becomes our identity. However, we are given a renewed mind (Romans 12:1-2) and we are cleansed wholly!

JESUS' BIRTH

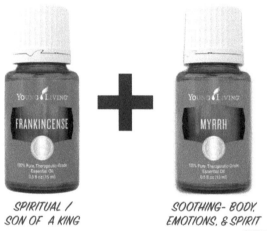

SPIRITUAL /
SON OF A KING

SOOTHING- BODY,
EMOTIONS, & SPIRIT

OilyApp.com- for iOS + Android. Download for graphics + videos + a pocket
reference on your phone. Young Living approved. 100% compliant, 200% awesome.

The birth of Jesus is highlighted by the unique gifts the magi brought to Him. One was the same oil used to anoint all newborn sons of kings in the ancient world- and was the "go to" for healing (Frankincense). The other brings peace and comfort to the body, soul, and spirit (Myrrh). Is this not what Jesus came to do?

* Next Steps

Now, you need to acquire the tools to get started. We suggest you order Young Living's Premium Starter Kit (it's an amazing value- it comes with 11 essential oils, a diffuser, and several other items!). You will eventually want the *Twelve Oils of Ancient Scripture* package, too.

If you're able to acquire these at the same time, do so! If not, order the Premium Starter Kit right

> YOU NEED TO ACQUIRE THE TOOLS TO GET STARTED.

away- and set an Essential Rewards order for the *Oils of Ancient Scripture* to come to you next month. (Essential Rewards is a non-obligation, non-contract program that gives you discounted shipping and points back which you can use for free products. We don't buy anything unless we do it on this program- we love free stuff!).

PREMIUM STARTER KIT
5 OILS
6 BLENDS
DIFFUSER
OTHER BONUSES

If you're waiting to get the *Oils of Ancient Scripture* (you'll want to order the other kit *first*, so that you receive the 24% discount on the Twelve Oils kit!), place it on Essential Rewards now and it will ship in approximately 30 days, giving you time to learn the first set of oils. (By placing the order on Essential Rewards, you earn points towards future *free* products!)

To place your order, consult with the person who gave you this material if they are a business-building distributor with Young Living Essential Oils. You will need their coupon code to receive the wholesale discount!

If they are not a distributor OR if you found this info on your own, *please go to* facebook.com/OilyApp *and send a PM, or connect through Instagram @OilyApp.*

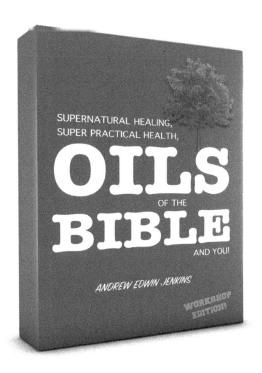

WANT TO LEARN MORE ABOUT THE OILS OF ANCIENT SCRIPTURE AND HOW THEY CAN HELP YOU LIVE YOUR BEST LIFE NOW?

Go to www.TheHealingWorkshop.info or search for the *Oils of the Bible* book on Amazon.

There are hundreds of references to oils throughout the Bible. In fact, once you "see" it, you might wonder how you missed it for so long. We see them mentioned more than baptism + communion combined!

Yet, we rarely see them discussed in a "church" setting.

Why did the magi brought Jesus Gold, Frankincense, and Myrrh?

And what did Jesus mean when He told the disciples to go "anoint with oil and heal" and then to declare that the Kingdom was now present?

And how do miracles fit together with health?

I mean, if Jesus healed everyone (which He did) AND if He said we would do greater things than He did (which He did) then why isn't everyone healed today?

If you...

- Believe healing power is available today and feel like God has tapped you to share His abundance & provision with others...

- Want a step-by-step process that's backed by the Bible, history, and science...

- Would love to give yourself and the people you love options when the miracles seem just out of reach...

- Think experiencing the Father's heart would be fun and invigorating...

- Just need some options yourself!

Then this book is just for you!

* OilyApp+

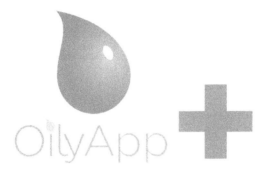

Want to watch the videos of this script? And other videos?

Oily App plus was created for you!

OilyApp+ is a web-based monthly membership / subscription service which provides you with each of the following:

- A monthly class- including a downloadable script AND the videos for the material in this book

- Graphics to match the class!

- 60 second videos to review each of the products mentioned in the class

- Access to Diamond+ leaders and biz-building tips

Here's a deeper dive on each of these features!

CLASSES

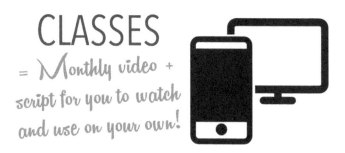

= Monthly video + script for you to watch and use on your own!

Monthly Feature #1 = An online class you can use to encourage, equip, and empower your team!

Every month- generally, the second week of the month- we go live and teach a class. Here's where it gets good… OilyApp+ subscribers receive forever access to the recording of that class, AS WELL AS the downloadable PDF or script we use.

Join the class simply to learn, or take advantage o the info by passing it on to others!

GRAPHICS

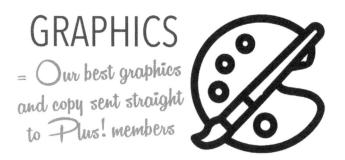

= Our best graphics and copy sent straight to Plus! members

Monthly Feature #2 = Our best graphics available for you to download + share!

We've pulled the best graphics and multi-pic posts from our Instagram feed and placed them where you can download them, then re-use them to share with prospects and grow your business. And, we've included our swipe copy in the files. Use it, edit it, whatever- it's there for you.

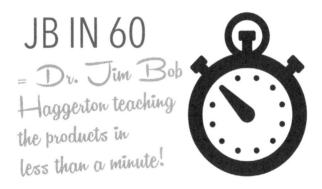

JB IN 60
= Dr. Jim Bob Haggerton teaching the products in less than a minute!

Monthly Feature #3 = How'd you like Dr. Jim Bob Haggerton to teach you about the products?! Done!

Specifically, he'll do it in 60 seconds or less. Whatever products we review in our class- be it the Oils of the Bible, the PSK, the core supplements... he'll give you the 60 second overview of each!

In the online portal, you can login and watch + re-watch as many times as you'd like!

BIZ TIPS

= Videos + more to encourage, equip, and empower you to grow

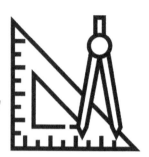

Monthly feature #4 = A recorded video call with one of the top leaders in Young Living! How would you like to hear how one Royal Crown Diamond hit the top rank without ever hosting a class- just by working through social media? Or, how would you like to learn how another did it WITHOUT social media?

What about learning leadership, work-family balance, gaining momentum, or finding your passion form others? Each month we feature a recorded convo from one of the top leaders teaching from their unique wheelhouse.

LEADERS

= Exclusive access to top leaders teaching from their wheelhouse!

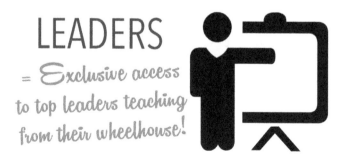

Monthly Feature #5 = Bonus videos and other tools we've created to make the biz super-simple and pleasantly practical!

You wouldn't dream of going to work somewhere without understanding how you get paid, and what you can do to make the most of your time. Somehow, we stumble into network marketing and forget to step back and ask those same questions, though.

Each month, we'll drop a resource about the comp plan, about teaching the business, or some other aspect that encourages, equips, and empowers YOU to reach your potential!

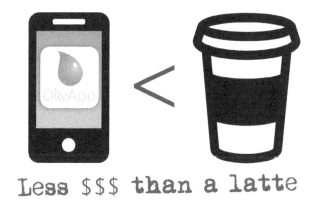

Less $$$ than a latte

You can find all of this our website- www.OilyApp.com!

And, it's affordable. In fact, it all costs you less than a latte!

In this book (and the videos) we talk about miracles and prayer and natural health- all in the same sitting. Some people think that to choose one is to negate the other- or vice versa. We've learned each of these things work together.

You'll find this book to be super-informative, as well as ultra-practical. And, we pull stories straight out of the Bible and show you the oils they used- and why...

We'll also show you things like...

- The guy most likely to talk about the power of the Holy Spirit (Luke) was also a doctor. And, the guy who healed a ton of people (Paul), also taught people how to be well...

- When Jesus sent the disciples out, He didn't just empower them to perform miracles, He also showed them to teach people how to be + live well.

And, we'll discuss rarely-talked about topics like anointing, laying on of hands, and other things we often overlook.